HYPERTENSION FOOD BIBLE

Science backed food guidelines, what you need to know about your blood pressure

WRITTEN BY

DR JESSE H. SEXTON

Copyright © DR JESSE H. SEXTON

All right reserved

INTRODUCTION

A balanced diet concentrating on normal consumption of fruits, vegetables, oats, nuts, lentils, herbs, and spices can be of tremendous advantage.

Contrastingly, excessive salt, alcohol, and processed foods may aggravate hypertensive condition.

Drugs, changes in eating lifestyle, and other lifestyle

adjustments can lower high blood pressure, while reducing the chances of developing related conditions. Hypertension increases the chances of a person to heart disease, stroke, and kidney disease.

Blood pressure implies to the power that blood applies to the walls of the artery as it moves through them.

In a perfect world, an individual's systolic blood pressure ought to be under 120 and their diastolic blood pressure under 80.

Hypertension begins when the systolic, or upper number, is somewhere in the range of 130 and 139 or the diastolic, or lower number, is somewhere in the range of 80 and 89.

CHAPTER ONE: HYPERTENSION (HIGH BLOOD PRESSURE)

There are approaches to overseeing hypertension. The condition doesn't frequently cause side effects; however, standard screening can assist an individual with knowing whether preventive measures are vital.

The U.S Preventive Service Task Force (USPSTF) gauges that

hypertension influences around 45% of grown-ups in the U.S.

The heart is a muscle that siphons blood around the body. As it moves, the blood conveys oxygen to the body's imperative organs.

Once in a while, an issue in the body makes it harder for the heart to siphon blood. For instance, this could happen on the off chance that the artery turns out to be excessively thin.

Steady hypertension can overwhelm the walls of the arteries. This can prompt different medical conditions, some of which can undermine life.

High blood pressure can be categorized into two (2):

Primary hypertension

This is likewise called fundamental hypertension. It is called this when there is no known reason for your hypertension.

This is the most well-known kind of hypertension. This kind of pulse normally requires numerous years to create.

It is most likely a consequence of your way of life, climate, and how your body changes as you age.

Secondary hypertension

This is the point at which a medical condition or medication is causing your hypertension.

If blood pressure is excessively high for a long time, it can cause serious damage to the blood vessels.

This can prompt diverse complications, some of which can pose a threat to one's existence.

The unit of measurement of the blood pressure is in millimeters of mercury (mm Hg).

Diagnosis of high blood pressure

One of the critical tests that has become a usual ritual at every visit of a doctor is the blood pressure with the aid of the monitor.

The nurse will wrap the band around your arm, which is

attached to a meter and a small pump.

The pump will be squeezed, which will lead to a tight feeling around the arm. Then there will be a pause to read the meter.

Dual numbers will be seen on the screen of the meter, for the blood pressure.

The upper number is the systolic reading, which is the highest blood pressure when your heart contracts to pump out blood.

The lower number is the diastolic pressure when the heart is taking in blood.

- Normal blood pressure is not up to 120 on top and not up to 80 below.

- Prehypertension levels ranges between 120-139 on top and between 80-89 below.

- High blood pressure, stage 1 is between 140-159 on top and between 90-99 below.

- High blood pressure, stage 2 can be greater than or equal to 160 on top and can be greater than or equal to 100 below.

The higher the blood pressure, the more regular and consistent the medical check-up should be.

After the clocking the age of 18years, the blood pressure needs to be checked at least once every two years.

But such individual has had high blood pressure in the past years, it should be checked, more often that stated.

Due to hormonal imbalance, there exist a divergence in the tendency for high blood pressure, but in males and females.

Conditions that can trigger an increase in the chances of high blood pressure in females include:

- pregnancy

- menopause

- using birth control pills

In the course of pregnancy, preeclampsia, a likely harmful condition that can affect both the mother and the baby, can trigger the increase in the blood pressure.

Thus, during pregnancy regular health check-up is crucial.

Obesity and diabetes can increase the blood pressure in children. Other causes include:

- a growth (malignant or benign)

- heart problems

- kidney problems

- obstructive sleep apnea

- a rheumatologic disorder

- thyroid problems

- a genetic condition, such as Cushing's syndrome

- the use of certain drugs

- a diet high in fat and salt

Unlike adults, high blood pressure is not usually connected with symptoms in children.

Examples of such symptoms in case they surface include:

- a headache

- fatigue

- mental changes

- vomiting

These symptoms are not unconnected to severe hypertension.

They may also show signs of another ailment or medical condition.

Newborn babies and very young babies can at times have high blood pressure due to an health condition, such as: kidney or heart disease.

In addition to high blood pressure, an infant may also experience:

- seizures

- irritability

- tiredness

- inability to feed properly

- fast breathing

- apnea

Other symptoms will be attributed to the condition causing the high blood pressure.

Below are some of the tests that can help ascertain a diagnosis. They include:

- Urine and blood tests

  These can look for underlying problems - urine infection or kidney damage.

- Exercise stress test

  A medical practitioner will determine an individual's blood pressure before, during, and after using a stationary bicycle.

The results can give a glimpse about the health condition of the heart.

. Electrocardiogram (EKG)

An EKG accesses the electrical impulses in the heart. For a person with high blood pressure and high cholesterol levels, the doctor may order an EKG as a premise for comparing future results.

Changes in future results might indicate that a coronary artery disease is emanating or that the heart wall is thickening.

- Holter monitoring

For a period of 24 hours, the individual carries the EKG portable device that is attached to their chest through electrodes.

This device can give an overview of the electrical

impulses in the heart throughout the day and indicates how it changes as the level of activity changes.

Modern medicine for treating high blood pressure include:

- Angiotensin converting enzyme inhibitors
- Calcium channel blockers
- Thiazide diuretics
- Beta-blockers
- Renin inhibitors
- Healthy Diet

The first five drugs although effective, has 1 or 2 side effects. The essence of this book is centred on healthy diets that can bring down the blood pressure if it is high or maintain a normal blood pressure.

Risk factors

High blood pressure can be traceable to certain risk factors which include:

- Age

The risk chances increase with age, because the blood vessels become less flexible unlike before.

- Family history and genetic factors

Individuals closely related to family members that are hypertensive, are more likely to develop it.

- Obesity and having excess weight

High blood pressure is highly probably in individuals that are obese or over-weight.

• Lack of regular exercise and body fitness

The absence of regular exercise and periodic visitation of gyms, will increase the chances and likelihood for high blood pressure.

• Smoking

When an individual engages in smoking, the available are for blood to flow in the vessels reduces, and the blood pressure increases.

The act of smoking lowers the level of oxygen in the blood, putting more pressure on the heart to pump faster, and also creating a corresponding increase in the blood pressure.

- High Alcohol intake

  Increase in blood pressure and other related complications such as heart disease, are the aftermath results of high alcohol consumption.

- Diet

  A diet rich in unsaturated fat, trans fat and salt increases the chances of high blood pressure.

More than half of the people with high blood pressure have high cholesterol.

The consumption of non-nutritious fats can lead to the accumulation of cholesterol (low density lipoprotein) in the arteries.

- Mental stress

Stress can have a negative impact on the blood pressure, especially when it is severe and persistent. It can occur due to societal, economic and psychological factors.

- Diabetes

High blood pressure usually takes place alongside with diabetes. Nonetheless, adopting a treatment plan to manage the disease can reduce the risk.

Black Americans are more likely by 40% to have hypertension and 30% Black Americans are more probable to die of heart disease than white Americans, according to studies.

A study conducted in 2018 further elucidates that, unequal access to excellent cardiovascular healthcare services is chiefly responsible this.

When to consult a doctor

Countless number of people that are hypertensive don't show symptoms.

In view of this, it is advisable for them to go through regular screenings, particularly, those with a higher risk.

The USPSTF advices yearly screening for:

- adults that are at least 40 years in age

- those with a high risk of hypertension

- individuals with a higher risk, including those who:

- ₒ have high to typical blood pressure: 130–139 to 80–89 mm Hg

- ₒ are obese or with excess weight

- ₒ are Black

Adults within the age range of 18–39 years, whose blood pressure is typical (less than 130/85 mm Hg) and who do not have other risk factors should have additional screenings every 3–5 years.

If rescreening by the doctor shows that blood pressure has increased, the USPSTF (United States Preventive Services Task Force) advices using an emergency blood pressure monitor for 24 hours to ascertain the blood pressure further.

If this persistently shows high blood pressure, the doctor will diagnose hypertension.

However, the USPSTF does not presently recommend scheduled screening for those aged 17 years and under.

High blood pressure is a highly hazardous condition, that is often not connected with symptoms, but can result to a heart attack, stroke, and other life-threatening conditions.

CHAPTER TWO: FOODS THAT CAN TRIGGER THE BLOOD PRESSURE

Peculiar eating traits, including excessive intake of red meat, alcohol or saturated fat, may likely step-up an individual's blood pressure state.

Ensuring a consistent consumption of a balanced meal can assist in the management and prevention of high blood pressure.

A diet consisting of all the classes of food can be from a plant source, unsaturated fats and whole grains.

Putting other indices in place, these foods can help in the management of the blood pressure.

Virtually half of the entire adults in the U.S are hypertensive, which will make them susceptible to stroke, heart disease and other health conditions.

Foods such as caffeinated drinks, baked goods, soda and many packaged foods that are high in salt concentration or sugar, can increase the blood pressure.

Replacing or substituting these foods in the diet can assist in bringing down or managing the high blood pressure.

To effectively handle and manage high blood pressure, the place of healthy diet consumption cannot be overemphasized.

Food materials that are high in sugar and sodium should be avoided, since they are the major accelerator of the blood pressure status.

In other to ensure a well-managed blood pressure, and to ensure a health condition that functions well, below are list of food that can step up the blood pressure, which one should be careful and mindful about:

1. Table Salt

In the event that you are attempting to follow a low-sodium diet, this appears to be an undeniable one, however it should be said. A good number of individuals go after the salt shaker by propensity while planning dinners and bites, yet it ought to be exceptionally restricted or stayed away from through and through while managing hypertension.

Track down new flavors and spices to use to enhance dishes.

2. Particular Condiments and Sauces

While supplanting table salt, don't fall into the snare of subbing specific sauces, all things considered.

Things like ketchup, soy sauce, salad dressing, grill sauce, and steak sauce all have a ton of sodium in them. Different spots where salt can be covered up are in pasta sauce and sauce.

Get to know various spices and flavors to add flavor to foods, all things considered.

3. Foods with Saturated and Trans Fat

There are unsaturated fats you can have in your eating routine even with hypertension;

however, saturated and trans fats are not among them.

Things seared in a ton of oils or meats that have a great deal of fat are terrible for both circulatory strain and cholesterol.

Lessen or dispose of red meat utilization. Assuming you really do eat red meat, ensure you read marks and pick the most slender cuts conceivable.

On the off chance that you consume a ton of dairy, change to low-fat forms. Also, watch out for cheeses with a high salt content.

4. Fried Food

Seared food sources contain a great deal of saturated fat and salt, the two of which you ought to stay away from when you have hypertension.

Barbecuing, baking, and sautéing are great options in

contrast to broiling. Air-fryers have become famous and are a decent choice as long as you focus on the salt substance of what you're cooking.

Any sort of breading or preparing blends ought to be low sodium.

5. Fast Food

On the off chance that you're observing any sort of nourishing rules, inexpensive food is an ill-conceived notion all-around.

A great deal of the food served at drive-through eateries is handled and frozen, then, at that point, cooked by broiling or cooking in high-fat oils.

Moreover, they are frequently vigorously salted. Since these are food varieties that increase the pulse rate, it ought to be kept away from them.

6. Canned, Frozen, and Processed Foods

These food varieties can be advantageous; notwithstanding, a considerable number of them contain a lot of added salt to protect flavor through the canning, bundling, or freezing process.

• Canned soups are top wrongdoers. In the event that you end up longing for soup, consider making your own with a low sodium recipe or search for low- and diminished-sodium canned choices.

This incorporates bundled stocks.

• Tomatoes and tomato-based sauces likewise have a ton of added salt when they arrive in a can or shake. Low-sodium assortments are accessible or utilize new tomatoes.

• A typical offender for high sodium among frozen foods is frozen pizza. Frozen pizzas with thick hulls and bunches of garnishes are particularly high in sodium.

• Frozen fish and meats may likewise have added salt.

7. Deli Meats and Cured Meats

Another food brimming with sodium is store meat. Lunch meats are frequently protected, restored, or prepared with salt, making them high in sodium. Relaxed meats like bacon are forbidden as well.

8. Salted Snacks

Numerous wafers, chips, and even desserts, like treats, are bad choices. Different things to pay special attention to incorporate jerky and nuts.

Those could seem like better snacks since they are wellsprings of protein and solid fats (in specific nuts); however, for those with hypertension, they can be awful information. Search for assortments that have no or very little salt added. Another great choice in the event that you are needing a crunchy nibble is popping your own plain popcorn and adding (without salt) flavors to it yourself.

You ought to likewise stay away from cured food sources, which are in many cases loaded with salt because of the pickling system.

Most pickling processes utilize a great deal of salt in the saline solution blend to kill microbes, and the sodium keeps close by after the pickling is finished.

9. Caffeine

Espresso, tea, caffeinated beverages, and soft drinks all contain caffeine, which is known to increment pulses.

Individuals with hypertension ought to restrict their caffeine consumption. On the off chance that you are an espresso sweetheart, have a go at changing to half-caff espresso, or decaf, in the event that you can't surrender it totally.

There are additionally without caffeine teas accessible, and certain assortments of tea have extremely low measures of caffeine normally.

10. Alcohol

Modest quantities of liquor have been found to bring down circulatory strain, yet drinking an excessive amount can increment it.

Having beyond what three beverages in a sitting can spike pulses, and routine drinking can cause enduring circulatory strain issues.

Liquor additionally cooperates gravely with specific pulse drugs.

11. Soda

Alongside the caffeine referenced above, soft drinks are loaded with handled sugar and void calories.

Drinks with high sugar content are connected to expanded paces of weight for individuals, everything being equal.

Also, individuals who are overweight or corpulent are at a more serious risk of developing hypertension.

Ladies ought to restrict added sugar to 24 grams each day, and men ought to just have 36 grams each day, probably, as suggested by the American Heart Association.

Meal Plan

For instance, an individual can eat the accompanying food varieties over the course of the day:

• **Breakfast:** entire grain toast with leafy foods, a glass of milk, or cereal with a natural product

• **Lunch:** barbecued chicken with a side plate of mixed greens or a bowl of quinoa and a serving of natural products

• **Nibble:** natural product, vegetables, cheddar, entire grain pasta or bread, or a food grown from the ground smoothie

• **Supper:** entire grain pasta, eggs, and a vegetable or natural product, or nuts with lean meat, like turkey or fish, and a couple of organic product sides

Daily habits

Way of life changes, for example, the accompanying can assist with bringing down the pulse and further develop heart wellbeing:

• stopping smoking, if material

• putting forth attempts to reach or keep a moderate weight

• tracking down sound ways of overseeing pressure, like contemplation and journaling

An individual ought to likewise

get sufficient activity whenever the situation allows.

Certain individuals might profit from beginning little and step by step stirring up to greater movement.

Individuals may likewise wish to find out if circulatory strain medicine might be helpful for them.

CHAPTER THREE: FOODS THAT LOWERS THE BLOOD PRESSURE

Taking diets that are healthy to the heart may also help in lowering the blood pressure and moderating it.

Eating foods that area rich in potassium and magnesium, may also be helpful in this regard.

One of the most common preventable risk factors for

heart disease is Hypertension. A very large percentage of people world-wide are hypertensive.

Below are 10 ideal foods for high blood pressure.

1. Salmon and other fatty fish

Fatty fish are rich in omega-3 fats, which have tremendous benefits to the heart.

These fats may help lower the blood pressure levels, by reducing inflammation.

71 studies were carried out in 2022 during a research on the health information of 4,973 people, to ascertain the relationship between omega-3 fats from the diet or supplements and the blood pressure.

The greatest advantage for bringing down the blood

pressure occurred with a daily amount between 2 to 3 grams of omega-3 fats (about a 3.5-ounce serving of salmon).

Higher omega-3 fat levels in the diet, including fish, may also reduce the chances of high blood pressure in young adults with no record of heart disease or diabetes.

2. Amaranth

Eating amaranth which is a whole grain, may help reduce the level of your blood pressure.

Research findings have shown that diets rich in whole grains have chances of reducing high blood pressure.

You could also attempt these other whole grains if you don't have a flair for amaranth:

- whole oats

- quinoa

- brown rice

- corn

- whole grain bread

- whole wheat pasta

A review was carried out on 28 studies and it was discovered that every 30-gram rise in daily whole grains consumed was associated with an 8% decreased tendency of high blood pressure.

Amaranth is a whole grain that's specifically high in magnesium. 38% of the daily magnesium required, can be obtained from one cooked cup (246 grams).

3. Olive oil

Diverse health benefits are present in the oil from the fruit of the olive tree. One of which include the lowering of the blood pressure.

A review of the studies in 2020 discovered that, as a result of the nutrients and plant-based compounds in olive oil, which include: the omega-9 fat, oleic acid and

antioxidant polyphenols.

In view of this, if added to the diet, it can help to lower the blood pressure.

4. Carrots

Carrots, which are nutritious and crunchy are staple veggie in the diets of many individuals.

They are rich in plant-based compounds that are beneficial

in various health processes, such as managing blood pressure.

A study carried out in 2023 discovered that, the possibility of high blood pressure decreased by 10% for approximately every 100 grams of carrots (about 1 cup of diced raw carrots) daily consumed.

5. Broccoli

Broccoli has several health benefits to the body. The

circulatory system is one of the recipients of its health benefits.

For example, introducing this cruciferous veggie to your meal may be a good way to lower your high blood pressure.

Broccoli is rich in flavonoid antioxidants, which may be beneficial in lowering blood pressure, by assisting the proper functioning of the blood vessels and boosting the nitric oxide levels in the body.

A study that involving the data collated from 187,453 people discovered that those who eat four broccoli servings or more per week had a reduced chance of high blood pressure than those who consumed broccoli once a month or less.

6. Herbs and spices

A good number of herbs and spices have powerful compounds that may assist in lowering the blood pressure via the relaxation of the blood vessels.

Other herbs and spices that may help in reducing high blood pressure according to results and research findings from animals and human include:

- celery seed

- cilantro

- saffron

- lemongrass

- black pepper

- garlic

- onion powder

- chili powder

- oregano

- cumin

- red pepper

- ginseng

- cinnamon

- cardamom

- basil

- ginger

A study recently carried out in 2021, on 71 people with risk factors for heart disease unveiled that, seasoning foods with 6.6 grams (1.3 teaspoons) herbs and spices as enumerated above daily was connected to lowering the blood pressure after a period of 4 weeks, compared to lower dosages of herbs and spices (3.3 grams/day and 0.5 grams/day).

7. Beets

Drinking beet juice may be beneficial in the reduction of high blood pressure, both in the short and long term. This is not unconnected to the dietary nitrate inherent in it.

According to a systematic review conducted in 2022, the research findings indicated that, nitrate from beetroot juice lowers systolic blood pressure in individuals with arterial hypertension, but does not influence diastolic blood pressure.

Tips for use include:

- the drinking 1 glass of beet juice daily

- the addition of beets to salads

- preparation of beets as an additional dish

One (1) cup of raw, cooked, or juiced beets is equivalent to a serving of beet.

It can be inferred from series of research that certain foods such as: fruits, vegetables, nuts, and oily fish — can assist in bringing down the blood pressure.

The integration of these foods in the diet may result to enormous health benefits in the long run.

CONCLUSION

It is impossible for a single food to "quickly" bring down the blood pressure.

But, having a meal rich in nutrients such as: magnesium, potassium, etc., may help lower or maintain healthy blood pressure over a long period of time.

Drinking water won't quickly step down your blood pressure,

but, ensuring a well hydrated lifestyle is crucial in enhancing an optimal blood pressure range.

Water can assist in meeting your hydration needs per day.

If you are hypertensive, consider greatly reducing or avoiding foods rich in sodium, added sugars, and saturated fat.

You can also attempt swapping fattier cuts of meat for leaner ones.

Along with other modifications in lifestyle, a healthy meal can tremendously lower the blood pressure levels and assist in bringing down your risk attributed to heart disease.

A medical practitioner can assist an individual in making a plan entailing: exercises, food choices, and other measures to effectively manage high blood pressure and lower the risk of cardiovascular disease and other health related issues.

Any individual who notices their blood pressure is 130–139 and 80–89 mm Hg or above should speak with a health care provider.

It may show an underlying health issue, such as: hyperthyroidism or kidney disease.

People inquire from their doctor the frequency of blood pressure screening they should undergo, to know the factors militating against their blood pressure and cardiac health.